T0063155

Other books by Cathy Covell

*A Patient's Guide to Understanding
Myofascial Release*

Feeling Your Way Through

A Therapist's Guide to Understanding Myofascial Release

Simple Answers to Frequently Asked Questions

Cathy Covell

BALBOA
PRESS

A DIVISION OF HAY HOUSE

Copyright © 2008, 2014 Cathy Covell.

All rights reserved. No part of this book may be used or reproduced by
any means, graphic, electronic, or mechanical, including photocopying,
recording, taping or by any information storage retrieval system
without the written permission of the publisher except in the case
of brief quotations embodied in critical articles and reviews.

Balboa Press books may be ordered through booksellers or by contacting:

Balboa Press
A Division of Hay House
1663 Liberty Drive
Bloomington, IN 47403
www.balboapress.com
1 (877) 407-4847

Because of the dynamic nature of the Internet, any web addresses or
links contained in this book may have changed since publication and
may no longer be valid. The views expressed in this work are solely those
of the author and do not necessarily reflect the views of the publisher,
and the publisher hereby disclaims any responsibility for them.

The author of this book does not dispense medical advice or prescribe
the use of any technique as a form of treatment for physical, emotional,
or medical problems without the advice of a physician, either directly
or indirectly. The intent of the author is only to offer information
of a general nature to help you in your quest for emotional and
spiritual well-being. In the event you use any of the information in
this book for yourself, which is your constitutional right, the author
and the publisher assume no responsibility for your actions.

Any people depicted in stock imagery provided by Thinkstock are
models, and such images are being used for illustrative purposes only.
Certain stock imagery © Thinkstock.

Printed in the United States of America.

ISBN: 978-1-4525-8961-9 (sc)
ISBN: 978-1-4525-8962-6 (e)

Balboa Press rev. date: 01/02/2014

Contents

Special Thanks!!

First and foremost thanks to John F. Barnes, PT! If it weren't for you, none of this would be possible. There aren't enough words to express everything you have done for me by being strong enough to follow your intuition. Thanks for your love and your guidance.

Thanks to Valerie McGraw and Carol Bannister for your support with this book. Carol, thanks for helping me when I couldn't quite put what I was thinking into writing. Val, thanks for your endless supply of faith in my ability and for your support during the times I hit the stumbling blocks. You were a rock during the storms.

Thanks to Sandy Hilton for being a sounding board, an editor, and a resource into the world of publishing. Thanks also to Dave and Jan Frederick. I really appreciate all the help.

Thanks to Donna Killion for your compassion and support during my healing process. You've helped me more than you know.

And a big thanks to all the people in the John F. Barnes' Myofascial Release (JFBMFR) community who encouraged me to put my MFR chat posts together in one book.

About This Edition

This edition of *A Therapist's Guide to Understanding Myofascial Release* contains updated information, rewritten material, and corrections to copy errors in the previous edition. I worked closely with Joe Miller, LCMT, in producing this edition. Joe suggested manuscript and copy edits to the original edition of this book; I accepted the ones I felt maintained my original meaning and tone.

Joe brought a special combination of abilities to the editing of this edition. A licensed, nationallycertified massage therapist practicing JFB-MFR exclusively, Joe began his journey with JFBMFR at the Healing Seminar in 2002. He has practiced JFB-MFR exclusively since 2004.

Before becoming a massage therapist in order to practice JFB-MFR, Joe spent over 25 years as a professional writer, editor, and business and technical consultant to companies in the United States and Europe. His knowledge of writing and editing, of JFBMFR, and of collaborative work methods helped me make significant improvements in this new edition.

Joe practices JFBMFR in the Chicago area. He also continues to write, edit, and provide language translation services to clients. You can reach Joe at jlmsvcs@gmail.com.

Foreword

John F. Barnes' Myofascial Release is the ultimate therapeutic art. Therapists and patients first learn the work on a structural level. As they progress in treatment, they find great depth to the JFBMFR approach. As skills and senses sharpen, the therapist and patient become aware of physical, emotional, mental, and energetic levels. It is at these levels that true healing can occur, creating large shifts in overall health. The best results are seen with those who have had the courage to delve deeply into their own healing possibilities and to take leaps out of their comfort zone.

Cathy Covell is one of those therapists who have dared to explore the possibilities of healing. She has come through her own pain to find techniques that affect real change. Cathy has worked for me at the Paoli Myofascial Release Treatment Center and is a great therapist. The Myofascial Release Seminars teach therapists from all over the world a technique that truly has the best interest of the patient at heart. Cathy has excelled in Myofascial Release and has been instrumental in answering questions on the Myofascial Release Chat Line with clarity while also keeping with the principles of true Myofascial Release.

The examples and insights provided in this book offer help to people during their healing journey. Reading and re-reading this book—as well as reading my book *Healing Ancient Wounds: The Renegade's Wisdom*, and watching my videos *The Fireside Chat* and the MFR DVD set—will enable people to understand the JFBMFR process at an even deeper level.

I hope you read the examples in this book slowly and carefully, and approach the questions posed here with the intention of seeing yourself and your patients in a new light. Read the question at the beginning of each chapter and pay attention to your reaction to the response to that question. See if you have a particular resistance to self-treatment, or emotion, or unwinding. See if you can go more deeply into the feeling and move past your own restrictions to a new quality of life and health. Learning is a life-long process; it does not end. It is important to enjoy the journey. This book is a valuable tool in helping you along the way.

John F. Barnes, PT
President of the Myofascial Release Treatment Centers and Seminars
1-800-Fascial
www.myofascialrelease.com

Introduction

The two books *A Therapist's Guide to Understanding Myofascial Release* and *A Patient's Guide to Understanding Myofascial Release* came together as a surprise for me. If I hadn't been given quite firm encouragement by some fellow therapists and friends, these books might not have been published. Just for my own benefit, I started collecting these answers to questions I heard frequently; then they turned into chapters and books.

While working at John Barnes' Myofascial Release Treatment Center in Paoli, PA[1], I was asked frequently the questions that have become the chapter titles in this book. I started saving my responses to many of those questions so I could refer to them as needed; this book is a compilation of those responses. The questions came from patients at the Paoli Clinic, from patients receiving JFBMFR at other facilities, and from people considering getting treatment. Some of the questions were asked on the MFR chat line. Anyone can join the free chat line on John's website (www.myofascialrelease.com)

---

[1] The Myofascial Release Treatment Center in Paoli, PA has since been relocated to a facility in Malvern, PA

and ask questions or share information. This book is a direct result of my posts on the MFR chat line, my daily interaction with patients and other therapists, my own journey of breaking free of chronic pain, and my listening to and learning from John.

Two invaluable resources are John's DVD *The Fireside Chat* and his MFR DVD set. *The Fireside Chat*, a 75-minute discussion with John, provides an inside look at John's perspective on the principles and methods employed in his Myofascial Release Approach. This DVD was designed to help therapists and patients understand the Myofascial Release philosophy on a deeper level. It can also help your loved ones understand the possibilities of a better life through the MFR process.

My book gives general answers and explanations to some of the questions patients and therapists ask most frequently when considering or receiving JFBMFR treatment. For more thorough discussions of how JFBMFR was developed and of the healing process, read John's book *Healing Ancient Wounds: The Renegade's Wisdom*.

I hope the information in this book is easy to understand and helps you with your healing process. Enjoy the journey. Believe me, it's worth it!

My background with JFB-MFR

My road to discovering the benefits of JFBMFR involved my own physical pain and dysfunction. I know having my own pain has helped me become a much better therapist.

Many of my symptoms began to manifest while I was in high school. I began having problems with ovarian cysts and had at least one ovarian cyst rupture each year through my late 20s. During my junior year in college, I had surgery to remove my right ovary and a large cyst. After I graduated with my first degree and before starting physical therapy school, I began having back pain.

I have played sports all of my life. In college, I played volleyball and basketball and was used to having a very active lifestyle. As my pain continued to increase, I was unable to walk more than a few blocks before I had to stop because of pain down my leg and spasms in my back. I thought surgery was my only option, so that is what I did. I underwent surgery in May and started physical therapy school in August. After the surgery, I didn't have constant numbness, but I still had pain, spasms, and occasional numbness.

During physical therapy school, and for the five years after I graduated, I searched for a way to relieve my own pain. I tried everything I was taught in school, with little result, and then started taking continuing education classes. I focused on taking any seminar having to do with the pelvis or the back. I tried all the manipulations, mobilizations, stabilization exercises, and stretches that were supposed to help alleviate back pain. I was unable to find anything that gave me more than temporary relief.

Believe me, it was very frustrating to be a physical therapist that was in more pain than her patients. I was also frustrated that many of my patients continued to have pain after receiving treatment. I felt like there was something I was missing. So, I started trying alternative treatments. I had about every kind of massage available and also tried acupuncture. All produced only temporary benefits.

My good days were ones when I had a constant dull ache; my bad days were when my leg would go numb or I had a knifelike pain in my back. I was unable to sit or stand for more than 20–30 seconds without needing to shift my weight due to the pain. I was slowly giving up the things I loved to do, like playing sports and riding horses. I was told that my pain was due to scar tissue and there was really nothing that could be done to help with scar tissue.

Here I was, in my mid- to late20s and in constant pain. I didn't even want to think about what life would be like when I reached my 50s. It was very depressing and frustrating.

It was at this time a therapist colleague offered to treat me using JFBMFR. Honestly, I didn't really have much faith it would help, but I thought I would just go along with it. I didn't have anything to lose by trying.

Within three or four treatments I felt a significant change for the better. I will always remember the night I lay down in bed and was able to straighten my legs fully. Previously, I always had to sleep with my knees bent and my trunk turned to the side or else I would have too much pain. My first thought was, "Wow, I can put my legs straight without pain!" Then my second thought was, "Well, we'll see how long this lasts." I was so used to having temporary results I didn't think these results wouldn't last either. Well, it's been over five years now and I'm still sleeping with my legs straight!

To say JFBMFR has given me my life back is an understatement. I can honestly say that I feel better at 36 than I did at 26. Not only that, but I now have the knowledge to help keep my body in the best shape possible for the rest of my life.

After my first treatments, I signed up to take classes taught by John Barnes. I wanted to be able to help others the way I was helped. The classes opened up my life professionally as well as personally. I finally learned ways to help patients heal themselves. The whole body approach taught by John completely changed the way that I treated as a therapist.

I continued to take John's classes and also participated in a Skill Enhancement Seminar at his Paoli, Pennsylvania Myofascial Release Treatment Center. This led to getting a position as a coverage therapist at Paoli and eventually led into working full time at the Treatment Center for 2 ½ years.

Being able to work at John's Paoli Clinic was a huge catalyst in both my personal and professional growth. The experience I received helped me gain the confidence needed to start teaching a seminar on treating horses using JFBMFR.

In 2007, I returned to my home in Indiana so I could be close to my family and bring JFBMFR to the area. I continue to work as a coverage therapist in the Paoli Treatment Center, help at John's seminars, and teach an Equine seminar.

Every day I am thankful John followed his intuition in developing these techniques and shares his knowledge with others. I hope this book helps others have a better understanding of JFBMFR so they can progress along their path to healing like I have.

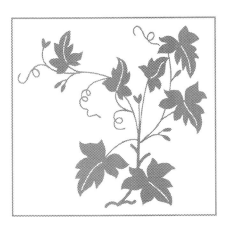

1
What is JFB-MFR?

I am about to give a very quick and limited explanation of John F. Barnes' Myofascial Release (JFBMFR). To get a more thorough understanding of JFBMFR, please refer to the many articles and books John has written. In these you will find the references to and scientific rational for true myofascial release. In this book, I hope to give you a basic understanding that can help you explain myofascial release to your patients and colleagues.

True JFBMFR is a full-body, handson technique developed and refined by John F. Barnes, PT. This technique releases the fascial system, a threedimensional web connecting and surrounding every system and cell in the body. To help people get the idea of the role of the fascial system, I like to compare the human body to an orange.

Outer layer: The thick, white, hard tissue that attaches an orange to the peel is similar to the fascia that holds the skin to our body.

Inner layer: When you cut an orange in half, the white fibers separate the different chambers of the orange. Fascia in our body helps to separate our organs and keep them in place. If it didn't, when we stood up, all our organs would drop down into our legs!

Cellular layer: When you look at an individual orange slice, you see the white fibers weaving throughout the slice, holding the slice together and also holding in the juice. Again, this is very similar to the fascial system holding our bodies together down to the cellular level. Our bodies are over 70% fluid and the fascial system is what keeps all this fluid (along with all the vital organs, nerves, veins, and arteries) in the right place.

Through trauma and repetitive motion or positioning (lifting all day or sitting all day), restrictions can form in the fascial system. These restrictions can exert forces up to 2000 pounds per square inch. This force can literally crush any of the vital structures near it. Since the fascial system runs throughout your entire body, these restrictions can cause pain anywhere in the body and compromise any system.

By "system," I mean vascular, neurological, muscular, reproductive, circulatory, digestive, etc. Fascial restrictions can cause digestive problems, fertility problems, circulation problems, neurological problems, cellular problems, muscular problems, etc.

These restrictions can become tighter over time, leaving you feeling like you are in a straitjacket and sending symptoms throughout your body.

JFBMFR helps to remove the straitjacket from the body. A skilled therapist looks at and treats the entire body, helping to restore balance. Releasing the fascial restrictions throughout the body decreases the crushing force of fascial restrictions, which in turn increases function, decreases pain, increases blood flow and nutrition to the body, and increases overall health down to the cellular level.

Fascial restrictions cannot be seen by x-ray or any other standard imaging technology. However, by developing sensitivity through taking courses and being treated, a skilled JFBMFR therapist can see and feel where these fascial restrictions are located. A JFBMFR treatment consists of engaging the barrier of the restriction and then waiting, allowing the restriction to release.

The barrier is the point at which the fascial restriction is in a lengthened or slightly stretched position. This is different from the end range of motion; it's more like taking the slack out of the system. Once the therapist engages the restriction at the barrier, it then needs to be held there for a minimum of 90-120 seconds before it **starts** to release.

For a good release to occur, the restriction needs to be held at the barrier at least 3-5 minutes. If the therapist holds the restriction at the barrier for a shorter time, he is not doing authentic JFBMFR and is not allowing the tissue to make a permanent change. Anything less does not involve the collagen component and works on only the elastic part—fascia is roughly 80% collagen and 20% elastic— and provides only temporary relief.

True JFBMFR is not forceful. The body is allowed to release, not forced to release. This does not mean the releases will not be painful. Pain and many other sensations often occur during a release. This is described more completely in the following chapters. What is important is following these guidelines when you are performing JFBMFR:

- look at and treat the entire body;
- engage the barrier and do not force though the barrier;
- hold for at least 3-5 minutes to allow for a true release to occur;
- do not force or lead the patient; and
- do not interpret what the patient is feeling. Each person's experience is unique to him or her.

If you do not follow these guidelines, then you have an incomplete understanding of the principles of JFBMFR. Some therapists take one or two classes from John—or take a class in school—and believe they are doing JFBMFR, but they don't really get the key factors. This is why it's important to repeat seminars and get treated yourself by a skilled therapist. If you have questions or need a reminder about something, remember the MFR chat line is a great resource, available on John's website at: www.myofascialrelease. com. This is a nice support system and a really good way to have questions answered and concerns addressed.

So, get ready for your adventure with JFBMFR. If you are looking for true, authentic healing, you have come to the right place!

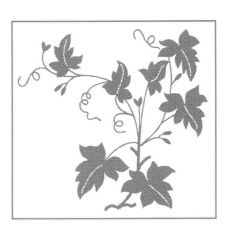

2

How is JFB-MFR different from other forms of therapy?

There are a number of significant differences between JFBMFR and other types of bodywork and traditional therapies. JFBMFR is a whole body technique that engages the fascia and follows what the body needs. Other forms of bodywork and therapies follow protocols and can be called "cookbook techniques." Many treat only the symptoms, try to segment the body, and ignore the power of the consciousness. JFBMFR therapists are able to tune into what each individual needs by going to the barrier of the restriction and waiting for the release to occur. Engaging the barrier and allowing the release to occur is a key difference between JFBMFR and other forms of bodywork.

Neither traditional nor alternative therapies hold at the barrier for sufficient time and therefore release only the elastic and muscular component of the myofascial complex. This is why these forms of therapy provide only temporary results. The JFBMFR approach releases the collagenous aspect of the myofascial complex, bringing about lasting results. The restriction needs to be held at the barrier for at least 3-5 minutes to allow the collagen to lengthen.

To illustrate this point, I like to compare two ways of stretching a rubber band. If you stretch a rubber band between your fingers, it lengthens. If you release the stretch after about a minute, the rubber band goes back to its original shape. This is like those therapies which hold at the barrier for only 30-45 seconds: all that is produced is a temporary result. The patient may feel relief for a little while, but then the feeling of that old familiar pull and pain returns.

If you stretch that same rubber band around an object like a book and leave it for several minutes, it will have lengthened when you remove it. This is what JFBMFR does: causes a permanent lengthening of the tissue. These rubber band stretching examples make it easy to see the difference resulting from holding the stretch for several minutes and to realize the difference in effectiveness is massive.

The awareness cultivated and used by JFBMFR therapists is another big difference between JFBMFR and other types of bodywork and traditional therapies. Feeling a restriction and holding the restriction at the barrier both require awareness. This barrier changes during the treatment as the fascia starts to release. You need to stay focused and centered to be able to feel the changes in the barrier, keeping at the barrier to keep the system engaged. If too much force is applied, the body starts to resist. If not enough force is applied, change occurs only in the elastic component, producing only temporary results.

It takes a therapist who is aware and centered to be able to maintain the barrier as the fascia releases. This is why it's important that you take John F. Barnes' seminars and receive treatment yourself. This awareness and feel cannot be learned through a book, and, as John says, you can only take someone as far as you have gone yourself. This is also why some therapists are better than others. Some therapists have gone to John's courses but are not able to stay centered. This makes it difficult or even impossible to feel the subtle changes that occur during a release. If you are having trouble with this, don't beat yourself up! It takes time for many of us! Keep treating, keep getting treated, and attend study groups.

True JFBMFR is noninjurious, results in permanent changes, and can help a person heal in mind, body, and spirit. The reason JFBMFR is noninjurious is due to the therapist's awareness during a treatment, to the therapist's ability to feel and not force the barrier. This is also what allows the full healing capability of the body to occur. The reason JFBMFR can help a person heal in mind and spirit is because the consciousness is recognized and enhanced. The awareness of the patient is very important in the healing process. This awareness is described more thoroughly in chapters 9 and 10, on feeling under the pain and on increasing awareness. All of these aspects taken together are why JFBMFR is called authentic healing.

3

Can JFB-MFR help with…?

Many of the questions that come up at the seminars, on the chat line, and in the clinic start with "Can JFBMFR help with [some diagnosis or another]?" At times therapists and patients both get caught up on the diagnosis. It seems the more specific or wordy a diagnosis, the more we doubt our ability to treat it. "I know JFBMFR is a whole body treatment, but can it really help with spondylolysis of levels L2-4 with radiating sciatica and plantar fasciitis?" I mean, surely with a diagnosis that long, it would take more than "look at the body and see where it guides you."

A diagnosis is just a naming of the symptoms. It is just a way to fit symptoms into a category so they can be "treated" or "fixed." The only problem is, as soon as the label is put on a dysfunction, the person with the dysfunction is already being sold short. What I mean is, when we as therapists are given a diagnosis, our attention usually shifts to "How can I fix that?" instead of "Where is the patient restricted or out of balance?"

Can JFBMFR help with every diagnosis? Yes it can. Am I saying that JFBMFR can cure every diagnosis? No, I'm not. But, as John frequently says, freeing the body from restrictions will allow it to function more efficiently, often correcting itself. Not only does this work with acute dysfunctions like back trauma from falls, motor vehicle accidents, etc., but also with systemic and chronic diagnoses such as high blood pressure, diabetes, fibromyalgia, chronic fatigue syndrome, and depression. JFBMFR can help those with chronic conditions peel back not only the physical restrictions, but also the emotions that hold the straitjacket in place.

Then there is the category of nerve/neural diagnosis: CVA, carpal tunnel syndrome, sciatica, etc. If the nerve has been completely severed, JFBMFR will not restore the nerve function. But again, JFBMFR can free the system so the available muscle activity will be more efficient.

Myofascial restrictions can simulate every symptom. Restrictions can compress muscles, nerves, and the components of every other system in the body. Age doesn't matter. Patients are never too young or too old to benefit from JFBMFR. Go ahead and give it a try. The least you will do is release some restrictions.

Trust yourself as a therapist and don't get caught up in the labels. If a patient's "symptoms" haven't changed after several sessions, change your perception. In the next session, let go of whatever you know of the patient's condition and history. Let go of all your expectations and let go of trying to "figure it out." Close your eyes, take a deep breath, and when you open your eyes again, use soft vision and just see where you are drawn and start your treatment there. Then just follow wherever the body leads. It really is that simple.

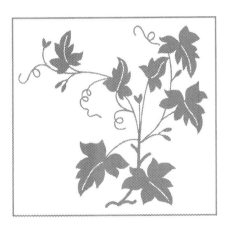

4
Will JFB-MFR overstretch the tissue?

Some therapists believe a patient with hypermobility must not have any restrictions. Others are concerned JFBMFR could overstretch tissue. Someone who has hypermobility can also have restrictions. Those restrictions might be contributing to pain and dysfunction, regardless of the hypermobility.

By really understanding the nature of JFBMFR, you will realize that when you follow the principles, the tissue cannot be overstretched or torn. Remember the principle of taking the fascia to the barrier and then holding it there. This allows the fascia to release; it is not forceful. To overstretch or damage tissue, a lot of force must be applied. Think of the rubber band example I used earlier. It takes a lot of force to cause a rubber band to break. You have to stretch it way past its barrier and all the way to the breaking point. Or, think of the amount of force required to pull a muscle. Usually a muscle gets pulled when a lot of force is applied with a lot of velocity, like pulling a hamstring muscle when sprinting or stopping quickly.

JFBMFR helps restore elasticity to the tissue by breaking down the scar tissue and adhesions that can form through trauma or repetitive positioning. Restoring this elasticity or "give" in the system actually will help prevent injuries. This "give" allows tissue to absorb impacts and to stretch instead of breaking when force is applied. Think of recurring sprains and strains. Why does the same area keep getting injured? After each injury, more scar tissue forms in the area to help prevent movement during healing. With more scar tissue, this area has even less ability to absorb impact or to stretch under force and so it tears again under impact or other force. Releasing the restrictions in such an area will allow the tissue to heal and help prevent reinjury.

5

Why would I treat somewhere other than where the symptoms are located?

Many doctors, therapists, and other health professionals are taught to treat symptom areas as a way to "fix" a patient's dysfunction. This seems like a good approach, but it really has not proved to be particularly effective. Instead of being taught to treat symptoms, the medical profession should be looking for the cause of the problem. Treating the symptoms—or masking them—doesn't help a person heal. It only gives temporary relief, if any relief at all.

If the philosophy of treating the symptom worked, people would be returning to a functional lifestyle without being medicated. Instead, people often receive a prescription for medication to mask the pain or dysfunction, and frequently live in a drug-clouded reality as a result. Even though this approach obviously doesn't work, many patients still believe the area with the symptoms is the area needing treatment. Sometimes it takes quite a bit of repetitive education to help a patient understand the need for the entire body to be treated.

The JFBMFR philosophy is to look at the entire being, instead of just focusing on where the symptoms are located. It may help to explain to the patient that, often, the area where the pain is expressing itself is the weak point in the system and not the source of the actual problem. Use the example of the pelvis being out of alignment.

Pelvic misalignment can cause the rest of the spine to be pulled off center. The body wants to be upright, so the trunk and neck will try to counteract the pelvic misalignment, resulting in a scoliotic curve. It helps to demonstrate this to the patient, using your own body in standing position.

When the spine is in its natural alignment, the muscles along the spine are not very active. This is known as the position of rest or position of efficiency.

These muscles can rest when the spine is in its natural position. When the spine is out of alignment, the muscles along the spine and neck have to work continuously and do not get to rest. This can cause soreness, pain, and muscle tension in these areas. Again, demonstrate this yourself in standing position; point out which muscles have to work harder when you try to stand upright with your pelvis off center.

When someone with these symptoms goes to the doctor, she usually gets a diagnosis which fits the symptoms, like neck pain, shoulder pain, or low back pain/strain. If she then goes to a therapist, the therapist usually treats only the symptoms, giving the patient only temporary relief or sometimes actually making the symptoms worse. To really help this patient, treatment is needed for the cause of the problem: the pelvic dysfunction. Then the symptoms and the dysfunction will both be helped.

You may also help a patient understand why you are treating areas other than where her symptoms are located if you explain to her that any diagnosis can have many different causes. For example, you could explain like this: "Let's say you have shoulder pain. The pain might be due to an actual shoulder injury; it might be due to your pelvis being out of alignment; it might be due to an old knee injury; it might be due to any number of causes. The only way to know is to look at the entire body as a whole, and to help restore balance to the entire system."

The best way to explain this is to have your patient feel her whole body connection during the treatment. During treatment, encourage the patient to sink into the area being treated; soon she will begin to feel sensations in other parts of her body. Leg pulls and arm pulls are an easy way to help a patient start to feel the connections. When you start to pull a leg or an arm, the patient often feels the pull into the low back or up into the neck.

It's quite amazing when your patients start to feel the connections. Remember, it may seem "weird" to them at first because most people have been taught the body is not connected. Soon they will start to feel even more connections and to realize how really crazy it is to think the body can be separated. This will help them start to feel the fullbody, three-dimensional web of the fascial system.

Have your patient remember this connection when she does self-treatment sessions. Let her know it's okay to start by treating an area that is hurting, but that while she is treating that area, she needs to feel the connections to other parts of her body. Explain that the places where she feels these connections are the areas she will want to treat next. Help the patient realize her body will actually tell her where she needs to treat. (See chapter

20, *Can patients treat themselves?*) This is when you start to help the patient feel like she has control over her own healing process. It's very empowering!

Also, encourage a patient to let go of any ideas of where she "thinks" she needs to be treated. Remind her just to allow her body to guide both you and her. Working that way, she will get the treatment she needs.

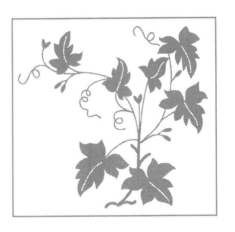

6

What if the patient's symptoms get worse?

Reproducing or flaring up symptoms—called a "healing crisis"—is a normal part of a patient's progression in therapy. It's good to start educating clients about this possibility during the first session. Don't tell them to expect a healing crisis; just let them know that soreness or an increase in symptoms can occur after treatment. Often, as we finally get to the bottom layer of the restriction, the patient will state, "I haven't had this pain since the initial injury."

Of course, the patient who is feeling those symptoms again isn't always as happy about it as the therapist. So, education is very important. Explain that this kind of experience is a *healing* crisis; it is part of healing and sometimes symptoms get worse before they improve. Patients often want to know why this happens.

One reason for a healing crisis is that the increase in the patient's signs and symptoms is his body's way of bringing awareness to the condition with which he deals every day, a condition he "tunes out" and doesn't feel. Another reason is that you are getting to and releasing the deeper layers of restrictions. Explain to the patient the layers of restrictions are like the many layers of an onion, and each layer will need to be released. Make clear ahead of time that as you get in the deeper layers, not only might the symptoms intensify, but other sensations or emotions might also surface. (Refer to chapter 15, *Why are emotions coming up?*)

Let your patients know a healing crisis typically lasts around 24–48 hours after a treatment, but it can continue longer. Again, you do *not* tell a patient he *will* have increased symptoms or soreness, because sometimes this does not happen. But, educating patients to the possibility of increased symptoms and soreness can help prevent some angry phone calls the next day.

Also, let your patients know the healing process isn't linear. At times a patient might feel as if he is taking two steps forward and one step backwards. Again, this is normal and it can occur as we go deeper into the restrictions.

It can be very scary when someone goes into a healing crisis. Always remind your patients JFBMFR is never injurious. Remind them to use the selftreatment techniques you taught them. A regular selftreatment program, combined with your therapy sessions, will help speed the healing process. Selftreatment also helps give a patient some control in his own healing process.

It may also help the patient to spend some quiet time bringing awareness into his body, especially into the areas that are speaking to him (i.e., areas that are painful, tight, etc.). Encourage the patient to try to sink deeper into whatever sensations he is feeling and then feel those sensations fully. Then, ask the patient to see if he can feel what lies underneath the sensations. Tell him to give his body permission to let go of anything no longer serving it and to give himself permission to do and feel whatever he needs in order to heal.

Doing this may bring up memories, emotions, shaking, sweating... the list could go on and on. The key is to guide the patient to let go and feel without any judgment or holding back. Help your patient understand that a crucial component of the healing process is *allowing* full feeling, and then clearing, of whatever comes up. Sometimes the purpose of these "flare ups" is to help the patient tap into something—an emotion, a belief, an awareness—that needs to be felt so the restriction can release and healing can occur at a deeper level.

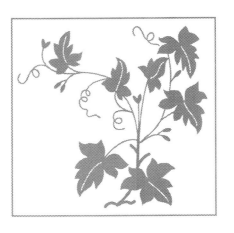

7

What happens when the patient's original symptoms improve, but new symptoms appear elsewhere?

After receiving treatment for a while, a patient may come to you frustrated by feeling "new" symptoms. For instance, her back doesn't seem to be hurting as much, but now her legs are suddenly very tight. Or, her neck pain is feeling better, but now she feels shoulder pain. Does this mean such a patient has new problems?

Actually, the layers are being peeled away and the patient is progressing normally. When the most prevalent symptoms start to fade (and this is a good thing!), other symptoms—ones that were always there but were not significant enough to override the major symptoms—become noticeable. I'll illustrate this using the examples from the beginning of this chapter.

The tightness your patient now feels in her legs was actually always there and was probably a result of bracing against the back pain. Legs often become tense and tight to help guard and protect the back. As her back has begun releasing, the tightness in her legs has become much more noticeable. The same thing is true for the example of the patient with the neck and shoulder pain. Once her neck starts to free up, the tightness and bracing in her shoulder becomes "louder."

When patients start noticing these "new" pains, use it as an indication of improvement. The area formerly the most restricted, the most "loud," has released enough that now it's possible to feel other areas in the body. Help the patient to see that feeling new symptoms is a sign of progress and a cause for celebration. The body is telling you where you need to treat next and where the patient should selftreat.

Now you start treating these new areas and see where they lead you. If the original symptoms seem to become "loud" again, then the releases have reached restrictions at a deeper level. You will start to realize the healing process is really quite simple. If you ever wonder where you need to treat, just ask the body!

8

Why does the patient feel sensations in an area other than the one I am treating?

When I hear a sentence start with "This is weird, but…" I know the patient is starting to have increased body awareness. Shaking, trembling, an emotion releasing, starting to be aware of the facial voice—these are all good developments. Like John says, try to get the patient to use the word "interesting" instead of "weird." People associate "weird" with something they shouldn't be feeling because it is a word used to judge what they are feeling. The word "interesting" comes more from a place of curiosity.

The body is completely connected with a threedimensional web of connective tissue called fascia. When you are treating a client's neck, he may feel a response or connection in one of his toes. Or when you do a leg pull, another client may feel a pulling in his jaw. When patients start to feel these connections, they often do find it "weird" instead of "interesting." Why is that? Because they have been told over and over that the body is not connected. Many health care professionals have been taught this too and it's what they tell their patients. Initially, when patients actually start feeling the whole body connection, they tend to doubt what they are feeling.

Your job as a therapist is to help your patients understand that feeling the connection is actually a vital part of the healing process. Encourage patients to feel the connections by having them keep their awareness in the areas you are treating. (See chapter 9, *How do I help patients "feel under the pain?"*). Once your patients start to feel the sensation or connection, ask them feel the sensations even more fully. Explain to them that when they feel sensations in an area other than the one being treated directly, this is the fascial voice talking. The body is pointing out other areas that need treatment. By tuning in and listening to this inner guide, they will be able to help with their own healing. The concepts of the fascial voice and of tuning in to see where to treat need to be reiterated when you teach patients selftreatment.

The next time you hear one of your patients start a sentence with the words "This is weird…", you'll know he has probably reached a new level of awareness. He has started to get the whole body connection and the fun is getting ready to start!

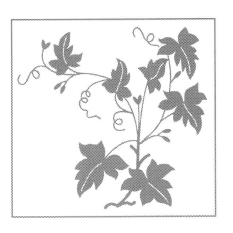

9

How do I help patients "feel under the pain"?

Over the years, most of us have learned to tune out pain or other uncomfortable sensations. To really get the most benefit out of JFBMFR treatments, the patient is going to need to do the opposite—allow herself to feel all the sensations even more, including the unpleasant sensations. These sensations can include burning, aching, tearing, dull or sharp pains, tingling, and shaking, among many other possibilities.

When a sensation is painful or uncomfortable, we want to help patients "feel under the pain." To do this, help your patients realize that pain and other sensations are just signals and nothing else. Suggest to your patients that they stop judging a sensation such as pain as "good" or "bad," and instead just let it be what it is:

a sensation. Suggest that they feel whatever sensations come up, instead of tuning them out, and then feel them even more.

Your patients need to understand that feeling a sensation is what the body needs to do to heal. Explain that a sensation such as pain is actually a signal trying to draw attention to something, and that, since most of us generally don't know what to do in response to that signal, we learn to tune it out. As a patient tunes in and feels pain or other sensations, she finally will be able to give her body permission to soften and let go.

One way I explain this concept to patients is as follows:

> Pain is just a signal. Its job is similar to that of a smoke detector; in both cases, an alarm system tells us something is happening which needs our awareness. The only thing a smoke detector can do is tell us there is smoke. It doesn't tell us whether some toast is burning (a mild problem) or the house is on fire (a major problem!). All it does is send out a signal, and then it's up to us to go see what is wrong.
>
> Pain is similar. It is a signal that tells us there is something we need to check

out. What we need to do is acknowledge the signal, and then go see what needs to be done. Feel the pain and ask the body what it needs to do. Sometimes, all the body needs is our awareness and permission to let go. Other times, we may need to make a change—stop the activity we are doing, selftreat, unwind, etc.

Many of us have been taught to ignore our pain or just to treat the symptom (block the pain). That would be like going up to the smoke detector and putting a pillow over it. Yes, you are blocking out the noise and keeping the smoke from getting to the detector, but you may then find yourself caught in a burning house!

When you feel pain, remember it is just a signal. Try not to judge it. Let yourself really feel the painful tissue. See if you can let it soften. If you are being treated, or are selftreating, and the tissue is softening, then you are doing exactly what you need to be doing. If the tissue is resisting, then you are putting too much pressure into the area. The body doesn't lie, so trust it.

You may find other ways to explain this concept to your patients. Just use what works for you.

A method I have found helpful in getting patients to allow themselves to feel is as follows. When a patient feels pain or another sensation, ask her to acknowledge that sensation, but then feel under it. What does the tissue feel like? Is it hard or soft? Does it feel like a rock, a steel cable, a sponge, something else? Can she breathe into the area? Can she connect with that part of her body at all? Have her describe that area and picture as clearly as she can. Then, have her picture that area softening and see if both of you can feel the changes.

Encourage your patient to tune in and notice even the smallest changes. If the tissue feels like a rock, can she imagine it slowly turning into clay or JellO? Have patients picture and feel your hands as they sink into the tissue. This is a release. Help the patient to understand that if the body is softening and releasing then it is doing what it needs to do.

The body will not release if it is being forced and it will not let itself be injured. This is an important concept, one which helps you and your patient during treatment, and also helps patients with selftreatment. A patient who is able to tune in and feel the tissue softening—even a hair's width—knows the body is doing what it needs to do.

It is important to help the patient realize that as a release occurs, the pain actually may get worse, not better. People tend to think the pain should ease as a release occurs. This may be the case at times, but at other times the pain actually will get worse as the tissue releases. Why does this happen? The pain may intensify because as the outer layers release, you are now getting down to the key restrictions and these are sometimes the most painful areas.

When you are working on a spot that is uncomfortable, notice how the patient often pulls away mentally and physically. This is a natural response to pain. Help the patient be aware of the pulling away, or guarding, and suggest instead that she breathe fully into the area and become as aware as possible of the area being treated. When the patient brings full awareness into the area, it will soften. Let her know that if the pain is intense, she can help the healing process by staying aware of the area as long as possible, pulling away whenever necessary, and then becoming aware of the area again. Taking this approach, patients start to feel how much more quickly the body releases when awareness is in the area being treated.

You may have to go over this concept many times during treatment. Make sure your patients know to ask for guidance when they need it. Then, remind them to quiet down and let themselves feel. Feeling is one of the key factors in the healing process.

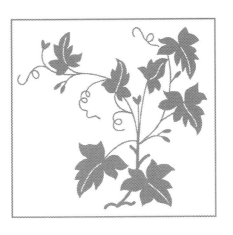

10
How do I help patients increase awareness?

When you first begin to dialogue with a patient, suggesting something like "clear a space" or "let it go," he may not understand what you mean. The following contract/relax exercise can help your patient increase awareness.

First, have the patient become aware of an area in his body that feels tense or one that is difficult to feel clearly. Then ask him to tighten that area and hold the tightness. Tell him to increase the tightness in the area as much as he can without causing injury. Ask the patient to feel the tightness fully and deeply and to notice how the tension spreads through his body. Then have the patient become aware of the struggle resulting from holding onto the tension when the body wants to let go. Once the patient has tightened as much as possible without causing injury, ask him to take a deep breath and let go of the tension, feeling how his body softens in response.

This is what it's like to let go or release. The struggle occurs when the body wants to soften, but the subconscious mind is telling it to stay tense for some reason. Sometimes the body just needs permission to let go and once a patient can bring awareness into the tight area, it will soften.

Sometimes a patient may have some belief or fear causing him to hold an area tight. In these situations, a person may feel emotions or have tissue memory come up during the release. Whatever the patient is feeling, just ask him to feel it even more and to give his body permission to do or feel whatever it needs to heal. Most of the time the body knows exactly what it needs to do; for that process to start, the mind needs to let go of control and allow the body heal.

Another approach that can help clear an area is having the patient breathe into the area you are treating. Ask the patient to breathe into the area your hands are touching. Some patients find it helps to visualize bringing a color or light into the area as the breath fills the area.

Just do some experimenting and see what works with each patient. Remember most people have been taught not to feel, especially if the feeling is uncomfortable. People may have difficulty at first with bringing awareness into a place that is uncomfortable or painful, especially if the area has been painful for a long time. Teaching patients to be present and aware during treatment is a huge key to their success in healing.

Remember that everyone learns differently. If a patient doesn't seem to understand one concept, just try another. Keep experimenting to see what works for each patient. Take the pressure off yourself. Just keep trying. If a patient is having a hard time with these concepts, encourage him to do some research for himself. Again, John's book *Healing Ancient Wounds: The Renegade's Wisdom* is a great source for any patient.

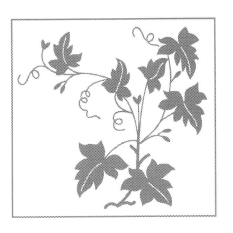

11

Why do I sometimes feel the same symptoms the patient is feeling?

A therapist sometimes feels sensations in her own body while she is treating a patient. These sensations may or may not be the same sensations the patient is feeling. The first time this happens, it can be somewhat alarming to the therapist. Sometimes the therapist is worried that she will "take on" the patient's symptoms or problems.

One explanation for this occurring is that your body is communicating with you and telling you where *you* are restricted and need to be treated. As John says during the seminars, when we are treating a patient, we are also being treated ourselves. When we are fully connecting with the patient during treatment, our own awareness level is raised. This means we may feel the places in our body where we need treatment. If you are treating a patient and you feel tension or tightness somewhere in your body, it means you need to treat that part of your body—that's where you have a restriction.

If your patient has an emotional release and it triggers you in some way, then the trigger is showing you something about yourself that requires attention. Notice the emotion you feel when you are triggered in this way and give yourself permission to go into and feel that emotion fully at a later time. Again, your body is telling you that *you* have restrictions (emotions, in this case) trapped in your body, keeping you from being fully present.

A second explanation for feeling sensations in your body while you are treating a patient is that you actually are able to feel being reproduced in your body whatever the patient feels. Sometimes this can be because you are not grounded; you can avoid this by doing some simple grounding exercises or visualizations prior to your treatment session. Grounding just means that you allow yourself to connect with a patient without feeling the need to "take on" whatever she is feeling. If you are grounded and you feel the patient's sensations in your body, then this may be how you are guided. You may

A Therapist's Guide to Understanding Myofascial Release

feel the patient's sensations as a way to guide you with helping the patient heal.

Most of us were taught we need to "fix" the patient. This sets us up for taking on the patient's sensation. We feel we are responsible for the patient's progress. In reality, all we can do is to facilitate the patient along her healing path; we can't do it for her. The following statement can help you become grounded prior to a treatment session: "Let me connect fully with [patient's name] so I am guided to where she [or he] needs treatment without giving or taking anything during the session."

You can use any statement that feels right to you. Some people use a specific prayer or statement. In this way, you can connect with your patient without "taking on" any of her sensations and without passing any of yours to her.

To be a good myofascial release therapist, you must let yourself quiet down and connect with your patient. When you do this, your endless mind chatter (consciousness) stops and you finally can connect into your subconscious. This taps into any of the physical or emotional sensations trapped in your subconscious.

Become aware of the sensations you feel. These sensations will show you where you need to do your

45

own work so you can be fully present for your patients during their treatment sessions. If we are not able to quiet down and be still ourselves, how are we going to be able to guide our patients in their processes?

12
How do I help the patient who has the need to "figure it out"?

Our patients often think they need to know why they hurt. Or, they believe what they are feeling should make sense. Or they think they should remember what caused the pain, emotion, or restriction. Some patients may say they believe they'll be unable to heal if they don't or can't "figure it out." Actually, the opposite is true. When patients are stuck in the mode of "figuring it out," they are limiting their ability to heal and let go. Reassure them that if they really need to know the cause of what they are feeling, the body will let them know. Then explain that knowing the cause doesn't really need to be part of the healing process.

I like to use the following example with patients:

Let's say you fell and hit your head on a chair when you were 3; you crashed your bike at age 10; you had a car accident in your teens; you slipped on ice when you were in your 20s; [add in surgeries and other traumas that led up to the present moment]. These traumas overlap each other and connect, like a threedimensional spider web.

When one restriction is being released, it may trigger physical and emotional tissue memory from multiple traumas. You may feel fear from the car accident, pain from the bike wreck, anger from your surgeries, and so on. All of these feelings can mix together and won't make logical sense at all when they all come up at the same time. If you try to figure it out by trying to identify the *one thing* that is the source of all these feelings, you will limit yourself to healing only one of these traumas. If you can give up your need to know and instead just feel each sensation completely, you allow yourself to heal multiple traumas simultaneously.

Just like the examples in John's book *Healing Ancient Wounds: The Renegade's Wisdom*, there are times during a release when the patient will know exactly what caused some restrictions. The patient will have very vivid and specific tissue memory come up. At other times, the sensations and releases won't make any sense at all to the patient. Let your patient know the releases he has without knowing the cause or source are just as effective as the releases which include a vivid memory. The important thing is that he allows himself to feel whatever comes up, regardless of whether it makes sense. Let him allow himself to be drawn down whatever path his body needs to take him. The body knows exactly what to do and where to go.

As a way to illustrating this concept, I like to use the image of drifting down a river on a raft, just letting the river take me where I need to go or just feeling whatever comes up. Most of us have been trying to swim upstream because we thought we "knew" what we needed to do and where we needed to go. Eventually, we get exhausted and we're forced to let the river take us where we need to go anyway. Why not just let yourself be guided from the beginning instead of waiting until you are broken down or exhausted?

The healing process does not need to be about struggling and difficulty; it can be about learning to trust our inner guide and yielding instead of resisting.

Help your patient understand the goal is to let the healing process be as easy as possible. Trusting yourself and being open to feeling—without judgment or the need to figure it out—allows the healing process to be much easier.

13

What if the patient has a flare up?

Often, patients are progressing along and then they have a flare up. (Of course, this goes for us as therapists too!). The flare up could be a healing crisis—things sometimes get worse before they get better. (See chapter 6, *What if the patient's symptoms get worse?*). It can be very frustrating when this occurs, but it is often part of the healing process. This phase has to do with the mind/body connection or the mind/body communication. During this phase, the mind and the body are trying to learn how to communicate with each other again. We have been taught to ignore our insights, intuition, or inner guide. When we do start to reconnect, it's not always a smooth or easy transition. The following is an example of how the mind and then the body might interpret this "flare up." I have found using this example can help patients understand the process more easily.

Here's the mind's prospective:

"Here I am progressing along nicely with this myofascial release therapy. The body is finally starting to open up. I can feel the shifts; I am starting to feel good! The body is finally starting to let me do the things I want to do! Then, I do something I think is very insignificant, like walk 5 more minutes or do a few extra household chores, and—WHAM!—that crazy body has a full blown flare up. I even feel some symptoms that I haven't felt in months. What is up with that!?"

Now, let's look at this same situation from the body's perspective:

"Here I am finally starting to get some release from the restrictions that have been crushing me. Then, that crazy mind decided to push me more than normal and I got scared. Why? Because I am finally starting to make some progress and that darn mind is trying to force me to do something that feels bad again. I tried to be nice and just send the ache signal, but of course the mind just kept on pushing. Well, I have learned over time the only way to get the mind to stop is with a full blown sensory overload. In other words, I'm sending out the full alarm, the full pain signal. And since the mind didn't listen to the warning ache, I'm even going to send the alarm to some areas that haven't needed it for a while. I have to do this because I know the only way the mind will stop forcing me is if I really send out the pain signal. I am tired of being forced, I am ready to heal!"

Over the years, most people have learned to shut down the communication between mind and body. We are taught not to show emotions, to push through pain, to discount our intuition. In this state, pain is the only form of communication that can get our attention. And we've gotten so good at tuning out pain that it has to spread and become more intense to finally get our attention. This is why patients may have a hard time letting themselves connect with the pain or other sensations they are feeling.

Through JFBMFR treatments, and with education, patients can start gaining awareness and thereby learn to tune into the body. As this new communication begins, it can be a little fragile and pretty combustible.

At times it might even seem like the mind and body are at war with each other. The mind feels the body let it down because the body can't do the things the mind wants to do, as in cases where patients have lost almost all of their functional ability. The body feels the mind has let it down because the mind keeps forcing the body to do things that hurt.

It's going to take time before these two systems trust each other again. In the process, there may be battles for control, with each side returning to what is familiar. For the body, reverting to the familiar will be sending out the full alarm to get the mind to stop. For the mind, it will be forcing through the signals. Mind and body will each tend to revert to those things which helped enable survival in the past. Helping your patient recognize these responses, and providing healthy alternatives, will be central in the healing process.

Emotions may also surface—feelings of anger, betrayal, guilt, etc. The only way the body will start trusting the mind to take care of it again will be by the actions that we take. Encourage your patients to go into these feelings and express them. Clearing these emotions is just as important as releasing the physical restrictions. Also, teach your patients to listen to the subtle signals the body sends. Teach them to take time to selftreat and really give full attention to the body.

As this communication improves, trust is established and the body won't need to send the full alarms. The body will start sending more subtle messages—like pressure or tightness—and the mind will now be open enough to feel these sensations and use them for guidance. Again, the key is feeling—specifically, feeling without judgment, feeling the sensations fully and letting them guide the patient where to go next. This may mean doing selftreatment, journaling, or feeling an emotion that has been ignored. As they do these forms of selftreatment, patients will be able to increase functional activities and do so with less pain and more ease. This is how we can help patients start to return to a fun and fulfilling life style!

Remind the patient to embrace the struggles and to feel the sensations. Both sides in the battle—mind and body—feel they have been wronged and both need some love, forgiveness, and healing. The end result definitely will be worth it.

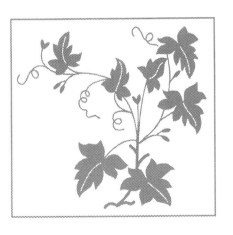

14

What if the patient has leveled out?

As you have probably heard or experienced for yourself, progression is not linear with JFBMFR. Sometimes it can seem like the patient moves two steps forward and then one step back, as described in chapter 6 on symptoms increasing and in chapter 13 on flare ups. The patient may even level out, reaching a plateau where progress seems to stop for a while. This might happen for a variety of reasons. Following are some suggestions you can give to patients to help them progress to the next level of healing.

1. **Have the patient treat places in his body that he does not normally treat**. Sometimes patients and therapists both get into a routine of treating where they *think* they should treat. As a patient progresses in JFBMFR, his body will shift and change. This means places that used to have the most significant restrictions have released, and now other places in

the body need treatment. Have the patient take out all of the selftreatment exercises and treat his entire body. You, as a therapist, need to look at the patient like you are seeing him for the first time. Get out of the pattern of treating where you think he needs treatment and ask his body for guidance. Treat him in sitting, in standing, or in other positions that you don't normally treat. Also, have the patient do some selfunwinding and let his body tell him where he needs to be treated.

2. **Have the patient feel whatever comes up whenever he is aware of the fact he has leveled out or is "stuck."** A patient may need to feel and release emotions to progress to the next level in his healing process. Encourage your patient to feel any emotions around this part—the leveled out or "stuck" part—of his process. Dialog with him to help him release any of these emotions.

3. **Have the patient journal**. Journaling can be a very effective method in helping a patient tap into his subconscious mind. Following are some journal topics you could pose to your patient.

    • Remember another time in your life when you have felt this way.
    • Start a sentence with "Right now I feel..." and just see where this takes you.

- Consider what you are gaining from holding onto this pain or sensation. (Sometimes people become so used to having a pain or a sensation that it can actually be frightening to let it go; holding onto it may be painful but it is familiar. Fear of the unknown can be very powerful. Ask your patient to consider this topic without making any judgment about whatever answer comes up. Suggest that the patient view this question as just another way to increase his awareness and to clear another level for further healing.)

4. **Have the patient get treatment by another therapist.** At the treatment centers, we treat as a team of therapists. Every therapist brings a unique style to treatment and we all have our own gifts to offer. Patients may need a variety of treatment styles during the healing process. Getting treatment from a variety of therapists is a very good way for a patient to receive all the aspects of treatment he needs. This will also help take the pressure off of you as a therapist for feeling responsibility to "fix" anyone. As a therapist, you will find it's good for you to exchange thoughts and ideas with other therapists and good for the patient to have the perspective of a variety of therapists.

5. **Increase the amount of treatment.** When a patient reaches a restriction that has been in place for a long time, he may need to increase the amount of treatment he receives in order to get to the core of that restriction. Once you get to the core layer of a restriction, it will release completely; until then, the restriction often tightens back down between sessions. This is why the intensive program is so powerful and effective: the patient's body doesn't have time to tighten back down between sessions and he is likely to be able to get to some of his core restrictions.

6. **Have the patient reread John's book and watch his video.** John's book *Healing Ancient Wounds: The Renegade's Wisdom,* and his *Fireside Chat* and MFR series videos, each have deep insights that can help every patient along his healing journey. The book you are reading just touches on the basics; John's book and videos are invaluable during the patient's treatment process (and in your continued growth as a therapist). Reading and rereading his book, and viewing and reviewing the videos, are priceless.

7. **Read other books on the healing process.** I have written another book called *Feeling Your Way Through.* It is more comprehensive than this one and will be helpful to your patient as he progresses

along his healing journey. You and your patient may also be drawn to other books to help your patient along the way. Peter Levine's *Waking the Tiger* and Colin Tipin's *Radical Forgiveness* are books that can be very helpful in the healing process. Authors of other books that may help are: Wayne Dyer, Caroline Myss, Don Miguel Ruiz, and Lee Coit, to name just a few. There is a wealth of information out there. Go with the books that feel right to you and suggest to the patient that he read the books that feel right for him.

8. **Have the patient take a break from getting treatment.** Sometimes the patient just needs to sit with what he feels and see where that takes him. This often forces the patient to feel some sensations that he may have been trying to avoid. A break will also give you time to let go of your need to try to "fix" the patient. That way when he comes back, you will be able to see him with a fresh set of eyes.

These are suggestions to help you along. The truth is each person's healing process is unique. The key is helping patients tune into the guide and the path that feels right for them. What works for you may, or may not, work for anyone else. Eliminate any preconception of how patients should heal and let them heal at their own pace.

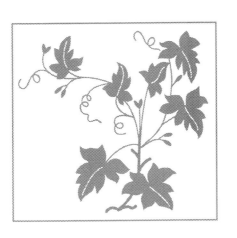

15
Why are emotions coming up?

During a treatment, all kinds of sensations and feelings can be released. This includes shaking, tremors, pain, and emotions. Why does this happen? This can occur when tissue memory is triggered during a release.

Tissue memory is a natural and normal occurrence. However, tissue memory often seems very scary and unnatural to many people. Most of us were taught at one time or another to believe it isn't okay to express pain or emotions. Any patient you treat may hold this belief very strongly.

I like to use the following example of tissue memory because most people can relate to it and it helps to show how natural tissue memory is. Have the patient think of a time in her life when she had the flu or was very sick. Then ask her, "What happened the next time you smelled or tasted the kind food you ate just before you got sick?" Typically, the patient makes a face and has some kind of tissue memory come up in reaction to this question alone. She will remember she had some sort of physical response to that smell or taste. She may say her stomach got queasy, or she started to sweat, and perhaps even came close to throwing up.

Explain that the response she had was an example of tissue memory. Her body associates the smell or taste of that food with becoming sick, and it doesn't want to be sick like that again. To try to prevent her from becoming sick again, the next time she smelled or tasted that same food, her body reminded her of how sick she had been the last time she smelled or tasted that food.

When this happens, the body is having a response to a proprioceptive trigger. Proprioception involves the five senses: sight, smell, taste, sound, and touch. When any of these receptors is triggered, tissue memory can occur too, as in the preceding example.

Another reaction most people can relate to is having a memory associated with a song (i.e., reacting to the proprioceptor). A person hears a certain song and she is "taken back" to a particular time in her life. Maybe it's a song she heard at a wedding, a funeral, or prom. When a patient's memory of an event is trigged, she may also feel emotions associated with that event.

I like to use these two examples to begin explaining tissue memory because most people can relate to them. Most people find the responses to the proprioceptive triggers in these two examples to be "acceptable" responses. Everyone's belief system is different, because we were raised in different families and cultures. Many people have firm beliefs about when and which emotions should and shouldn't be felt. Help your patient see how "normal" it is to have emotions triggered during a treatment session. Also, help her to understand how much her healing process will be helped by allowing herself to feel whatever comes up.

You can build on these examples as a way to explain why emotions may come up during treatment. Explain that when the fascia is released through touch (which is one of the proprioceptors), tissue memory may be triggered in the process. If an area being released was injured during a scary event—car accident, abuse, etc.—sensations that occurred during that event might also be released. Let your client know that: she might feel fear; her body might shake; she might feel the pain just as intensely as when the trauma originally occurred. She might feel any and all of the sensations that were caused during the trauma and that have been trapped in the fascia, and in her body. Actually, what is happening is she is becoming aware of what her body is feeling all the time on the subconscious level. Help her to understand that when this happens, what she needs to do is feel *fully* the sensations that occurred during the trauma; then those sensations can be released and she can heal completely.

Feeling these sensations *fully* is easy to say, but not necessarily easy to do. Remember the sensations can feel as intense as they did during the initial trauma itself. Many times the sensations that occurred were overwhelming, which is why a person wasn't able to release them in the first place. When we are overwhelmed with pain, fear, etc., one of our automatic selfdefense mechanisms is to leave our body. To "leave the body" is to become completely numb, pushing the pain and emotions below the conscious level.

When the tissue memory is triggered, the sensations that arise can be just as overwhelming as they were in the original trauma. Remind the patient that she doesn't have to feel it all at once. Encourage her to feel as much she can and to pull out of the feeling if it begins to be overwhelming. Let her know that it's okay to chip away at it bit by bit. The patient always needs to have the control over how much she feels.

As therapists, our job is to provide an environment in which it is safe for our patients to heal. For patients to feel safe, they need to know they can stop any treatment at any time. Have your patient say to herself, "I survived." Let her know she is safe now. Tell her it's okay to feel and release those sensations now, so she can live fully in the present; it's time to heal.

Again, let go of your intention during a treatment. All you can do is provide a safe environment for your patient. Let her know that it's okay for her to express emotions. If emotions come up, encourage her to feel them fully.

If you shut down your patient's emotional release, you will hinder her healing process. If you are not comfortable with feelings being expressed, you need to look at your own belief system and heal the part in you that is triggered when others show emotions. That way, you can fully be present and open for your patient to heal.

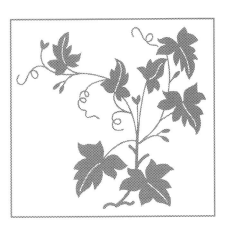

16
Why does the patient need to feel the emotions that come up?

Patients often start to have emotions surface during the treatment process. In fact, feeling the emotions can be a very big catalyst in the healing process. Why is it important to tap into and feel any emotions associated with our pain or injury? As we all know, stress and emotions can cause physical tightness and pain. It's important that we let the patient know emotions are normal and natural during the healing process.

You don't need to explain this during the first treatment, as not all patients will tap into their emotions. Use your judgment as to when it's appropriate. Often, those who have had chronic pain have been told the pain is "all in your head" and, with that, have had their pain completely discounted. Make sure you explain that the physical restrictions caused by traumas and stresses—physical *and emotional*—are real. They can be seen and felt, and they can cause crushing pain.

Almost every kind of chronic and acute pain has an emotional component. The emotional component might be fear or anger that occurred at the time of injury, or frustration and sense of loss of control that often accompanies chronic pain. If the emotional component isn't addressed, then the physical restriction will not release fully, causing continued pain.

As emotional pain comes to the surface, the patient may wonder why he would want to feel those awful feelings. Why not just stuff them down? Because beside the fact that he will not be painfree if he holds on to the emotions, he will not truly live until the emotions are cleared. These stored emotions are the cause our strong reactions to certain triggers. A reaction is just what it says: a re action. When someone flies off the handle, or starts crying for no apparent reason, he is reacting to emotions that are stuffed inside. He is trapped in the past, unable to truly live in the moment.

All of this became clear and real to me after I finally cleared the pain surrounding my dad's death. Before

I did this, whenever I would think of my dad, all I could feel and remember was the pain and grief that surrounded his loss. Now I can tap into and feel all the love and good times we shared.

By clearing pain and sorrow of losing someone close, we can reconnect with the love we shared with that person. By clearing our restrictions and letting go of the pain of the past, we can embrace fully the love and beauty of the present. The process may not always be easy, but it is always worth it.

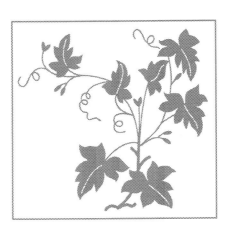

17

What if the patient doesn't want to feel or remember that again?

Patients often say they don't want to feel the pain "again," or that they have already "dealt with that" and don't want to remember it again. If a patient has truly "dealt with" an issue, truly healed, then it will no longer cause a reaction in her body when she discusses it.

Most people have "dealt with" past trauma by talking about it. This only deals with *part* of the healing process. A person truly heals only after feeling the pain fully—and feeling the other sensations associated with the trauma as well—and then letting go of all those sensations.

The fact is, on the subconscious level, a person experiences unresolved trauma all day and all night long, like a broken record. To the subconscious mind, the trauma is happening continuously. To this person's subconscious mind, the truck is about to hit her; the surgical knife is cutting her; she is still experiencing the abuse.

In the safety of the therapeutic environment, it is better for a patient to feel intense therapeutic pain, sadness, anger, or other sensations and emotions for a short time, then to spend the rest of her life "coping" with any of these. "Coping" is a losing battle; it is simply the subconscious mind exercising control by bracing constantly against the unresolved trauma. This constant bracing causes the ground substance of the fascia to solidify, which in turn forms restrictions. Over time, these restrictions will eventually worsen and spread throughout the body time. The end result can make a person feel like she is made of cement or wearing a straitjacket.

Remind your patient that JFBMFR never injures or re-traumatizes. JFBMFR allows for the discovery of unresolved physical/emotional trauma. The mind/body is then able to process this information through the conscious mind and complete the process known as release. JFBMFR allows for healing on the deepest level.

Let the patient know that she doesn't have to feel it all at once. Each time she allows herself to feel the pain/trauma deeply and then clears (releases) it, she will come closer to healing fully. Each time she does this, she will become lighter and become more herself again. She will be able to live fully in the present, without the present being a life full of reacting to past traumas. Again, let her know that she is always in control and can feel as deeply as she allows herself to do. Also, the more deeply she allows herself to feel, the more quickly she will be able to heal.

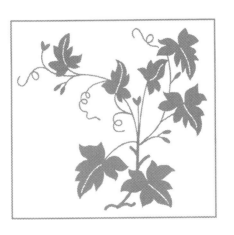

18
Why is the patient's body moving?

If a patient has read John's book: *Healing Ancient Wounds: The Renegade's Wisdom*, or has heard others talking about unwinding, he may come in with questions about unwinding. If a patient has no idea what JFBMFR involves, I don't bring up unwinding until he has either had a few treatments and is starting to get the whole body connection, or started to have some unwinding occur. It's much easier to explain something while it's occurring and the patient can actually feel it. The following explanation of unwinding seems to help patients. Just keep it simple and explain it more deeply as the patient's receptiveness grows. If the progression of treatment allows for it, first explain tissue memory and then unwinding; it's often much easier for the patient to understand tissue memory before understanding unwinding.

Remind the patient that his body is like a threedimensional web of connected tissue. Fascia is not linear and neither are releases. As the restrictions begin to release along this threedimensional web, movement might start to occur; this is called unwinding. Sometimes unwinding occurs in small motions and movements, and at other times, the unwinding can involve the entire body. It doesn't matter whether the movement is small or large; both are equally powerful. With any unwinding, tissue memory and emotions might come up. (Refer to chapter 15, *Why are emotions coming up?*) During any session, a patient might shift back and forth between being still—or having only slight unwindings—and having very energized unwindings.

Unwinding is the body's way of putting a part (shoulder, leg, head, etc.), or all, of the body in the position in which the injury occurred. Moving into such a position helps the body to achieve a complete release. For example, if a person hurt his arm while throwing a ball, the arm might move itself over his head in an unwinding until it reaches the position it was in when it was injured during the throw. Or, a patient might have been thrown from a horse and landed upside down. In that case, his body may need to reproduce the motion of the fall to release that trauma.

During an unwinding, the body will move until it gets back into the position of injury; that position is called a "still point." Then it will wait in this position, processing in whatever manner it needs to do. This might be through an emotional response like crying or moaning, through a physical response like shaking or sweating, or even through a feeling of calm. Once this still point is resolved, the body will move on to the next layer. Strong tissue memory often comes up during unwinding. The patient might have sensations come up that occurred during the trauma, as I explained in the chapter on tissue memory (see chapter 15, *Why are emotions coming up?*).

After that restriction is resolved, the body will move on to the next still point. This next still point may be completely different from the previous one; however, the body might return to the exact same position it was just in, while the patient releases at a deeper level. If the restriction was due to a very traumatic event, the patient might return to the same still point a number of times to release fully the pain and other sensations associated with that trauma. It might be too painful or scary to feel all the sensations associated with the trauma at once.

Every night while we sleep, the body naturally releases some of the traumas through dreaming and movement. The only problem is that the bed gets in the way! This is where you come in. The patient needs the assistance of a skilled therapist to help complete the healing process. The therapist's job is to help take the effects of gravity out of the patient's fascial system and to provide the patient a safe environment in which to release. You do not lift or move the patient. You follow the lead of the patient's body, helping the patient stay in any still point that emerges, until the restriction is released completely.

To understand unwinding fully, and to be able to feel comfortable during a patient's unwinding, you need to take the unwinding courses. Remember to watch the patient's body language and to do what the body asks. If the patient is reaching, then help him stretch by elongating that body part. If he makes a fist or is pushing with his arms or legs, then you may need to resist the movement. Just test the waters and see what happens. If you feel like you are working too hard, then you *are* working too hard. The body can do this with or without you; occasionally, it just needs some help getting into the positions it needs to be in so it can heal.

As with any part of the JFBMFR treatment, the best advice to give is "let go of the outcome." Let each unwinding be whatever it needs to be, whether it manifests as subtle (small) movements or as more energetic (full body) movements. Remember, no particular kind of movement is better than any other. Sometimes we think we need to have big motion and a lot of noise to have a powerful unwinding. That is simply not true. Sometimes, while the body stays completely still, a very powerful unwinding occurs internally. Don't try to force movement. Unwinding is more about letting go than about "getting there."

Before a treatment , it helps to remind the patient to let go of any expectations. Have the patient give himself permission to do and feel whatever he needs to do to reach his next level of healing. Have him let go of any preconceived notions of what he needs to do or feel. At the time of treatment, his body might need unwinding with an emotional release, or structural work, or any number of other things. Ask your patient to trust that his body knows what it needs and to take all the pressure off himself. If the patient lets go, he will end up getting exactly the treatment he needs.

This advice also applies to you as a therapist. If you think you know ahead of time what the patient needs, you really have no idea what he needs. Let go of any expectations about the treatment outcome or how you are going to "get" the patient to heal or unwind. You can't make someone unwind. All you do is create a safe space in which a person can let go. Then, if he needs to unwind and is willing to let go, he will do that. The same goes for healing. You can't make someone heal. All you can do is provide the opportunity for him to heal. So take all the pressure off of yourself and trust the patient's body. It's up to the patient to do the rest.

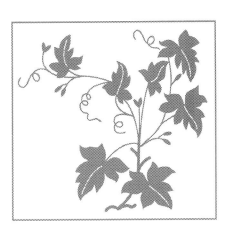

19
How do I dialogue?

The JFBMFR approach to dialoguing is to encourage the patient to feel as fully as possible whatever sensation or emotion she is experiencing at the moment. This means sinking into and feeling the pain, ache, tingling, sadness, fear, anger or whatever sensation she may feel. Dialoguing at appropriate times can help facilitate the healing process.

Dialoguing comes from a place of knowing, not doing, just like the rest of the JFBMFR treatment. You dialogue when you "feel" you should, not when you "think" you should. You will start to have words and phrases pop up in your head, just like when you start to feel guided to treat a certain part of the body. This is how you know you are being guided to speak.

When you feel that you should dialogue, remember the following guidelines. We do not lead or analyze; we guide. We *do not* tell people what is going on with them and what they need to do about it. Each individual's every sensation is unique. For example, what the color red means to one person could be something completely different from what it means to someone else. The color red might even mean different things to someone at different times.

Instead of analyzing, we approach the patient from a place of curiosity. We ask, "What are you feeling?" Then we wait for an answer. Be patient and wait for the answer. Never ask questions rapid fire. Ask one question and then wait. You may need to tell the patient to feel for an answer. If the patient comes up with an answer quickly, it's usually from her head and not from her felt sense. Encourage the patient to feel for the answer.

Here are some examples of dialoguing questions:

- What are you experiencing, sensing, or seeing?
- How does that feel?
- Where do you feel it?
- What does that mean or symbolize to you?
- What do you need to see, feel, know, or do to let this go and to resolve it fully?
- What do you need to do or feel in the next 5–10 minutes to reach resolution for this session?
- Who would you be without this pain?

Help the patient understand clearly that the answer might not come in conscious form, does not need to be understandable, and does not need to make logical sense. If the patient does answer a question you pose, continue dialoguing to help her uncover any meaning for herself. Again, *do not* interpret the patient's answer or suggest what it means to you. Do not tell her what she should or should not be doing. The patient's healing has nothing to do with you or your beliefs. Her healing has to do with her own interpretation of the insights that come to her during the treatment.

Remember that sometimes you don't need to say anything. If you are trying to think of something to say, it's probably best to say nothing at all.

It's a good idea for you and your patients to listen to John's *Inner Awareness* recordings. These are very helpful with dialoguing and with helping to bring in awareness during the treatment session.

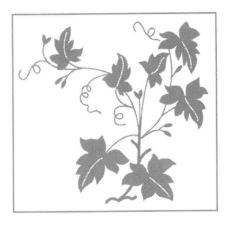

20

Can patients treat themselves?

One of the best things about JFBMFR is that you can teach patients how to treat themselves. You teach them they actually can have a major impact on their own recovery. In fact, you let them know you can only take them so far, and then it's up to them. JFBMFR is an interactive treatment. Let the patients know they need to be aware and present during treatments (as I've discussed in preceding chapters) and the more they selftreat, the more quickly they can progress. This may be the first time some patients have been in a place of power for involvement in their own recovery. Usually, patients are just told what to do or given pills to take. The following questions and answers may help you guide your patients.

- *How do I know where to treat?*

    Your patient can treat places where he feels symptoms and also places you suggest he treat.

Remind him that where he feels the symptoms may be different from where the cause of the problem is located. It may help him to tell him where you sense some of the key restrictions in his body. Also, have him just start stretching and moving and then see where he feels a pull or tightness. For instance, suggest that he reach over his head and start stretching like he does when he wakes up in the morning. Demonstrate this, and then do it with him; it can be really helpful. Have him move his body and just see how it feels. Help him to start becoming aware of how his body feels throughout the day and explain this will guide him to areas that need to be treated.

• *How do I treat myself?*

Part of your job as a therapist is to direct your patient in stretches and in the use of tools for selftreatment. We usually have patients use the following tools: small ball, foam roll, Nola Rola, Theracane, and Occipivot. With these tools, your patient can pretty much treat his entire body. The tools are a great investment and will more than pay for themselves with the relief they provide. You can purchase all of these tools directly from the manufacturer or you can order them from the Myofascial Release Treatment Center (1-800-327-2425).

The book *Myofascial Stretching: A Guide to Selftreatment*, by Brenda Pardy, OTR and Jill Morton, MS, OTR, is a very good resource for selftreatment. This book has detailed pictures of stretches and the use of the small ball for selftreatment; it also has some very good general information on selftreatment. You can order it by going to www.DenverMyofascialRelease.com or calling 1-303-649-9007. *Comprehensive Myofascial Self Treatment,* by Joyce Karnis Patterson, PT, is another good resource for selftreatment. To order this book, visit www.mfrselftreat.com. The *Myofascial Freedom* DVD by John F. Barnes goes through some the selftreatment ideas and can help you in guiding your patient's selftreatment program.

• *How do I know if I'm doing it right?*

This calls for awareness on the patient's part. Just like during a treatment, when he's selftreating, he needs to feel the area he's treating and feel the releases when they happen. As you know, it can sometimes be painful when a restriction is being treated. Your role in this situation is to help the patient know the difference between therapeutic pain and nontherapeutic pain (see chapter 9, *How do I help patients "feel under the pain"?*). Remind your patient that as long as the tissue is softening and giving—no matter how small the change—he is doing what his body needs. If the body is resisting, he is putting too much pressure into the area. Forcing the system will only cause more tightness to occur.

* *How long do I treat myself?*

Remind the patient it takes a minimum of 120 seconds for a release to *start* happening. He should hold the release for at least 3–5 minutes. Anything less will be a waste of time. Suggest he put on some calming music and hold a release for at least one composition. That way he will be holding the release long enough and won't be constantly looking at the clock.

* *How often should I treat?*

Self-treatment should become part of your patient's daily routine. He doesn't need to treat every area every day. As he becomes aware of the significant areas, he will realize where he needs to focus more of his attention. (Again, you can help him realize where these areas are located.) Consider his predominant posture during a typical day; this will point to where he needs to focus some treatment. Most people need to open up their chest and their hip flexors because they spend a lot of time sitting, driving, typing, etc. and these activities keep them in a flexed position.

• *What if I am sore after I treat myself?*

As long as he was treating with awareness and not forcing the system, your patient did exactly what his body needed. As with treatment from his therapist, he may have soreness or even experience a healing crisis after a self-treatment session. If he did force the system, then he gave himself a traditional treatment and he will have only temporary results.

Reiterate to your patient that the more he puts into his self-treatment program, the better he will feel and the more quickly he will improve. JFBMFR teaches you how to take care of yourself for the rest of your life. It helps you maintain a functional and pain free lifestyle; self-treatment is a critical part of this maintenance.

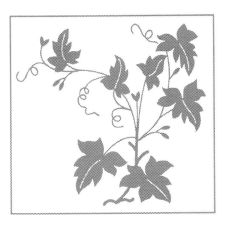

21
Will the patient need to do this forever?

The following questions about duration of treatment come up frequently. When will I be free of all restrictions? How long do I need to do the selftreatment? When am I done? Do I have to do this forever? My answer to any of these questions is the same: Do you brush your teeth only 2 or 3 times a week for 2 months and expect your teeth to stay healthy your entire life?

Most people have come to the understanding that they need to brush their teeth at least twice a day to promote healthy teeth and gums. This has become a habit, so it doesn't seem anything out of the ordinary. But, sometimes when you suggest to a patient that she needs to selftreat every day to keep her body healthy, she seems to act like you are asking her to run a marathon.

Use the toothbrush analogy to help the patient understand the need for daily self-treatment. Eventually, it will become just as much of a habit to treat herself daily as it has become to brush her teeth several times a day. When she is in pain, it will become a habit to grab the yellow ball, foam roll, or Theracane instead of grabbing the Advil. This is what it means to give someone the power to take care of herself.

When a person gets into the habit of treating herself, she will actually feel out of sorts when she doesn't treat herself. It will be like going a few days without brushing her teeth. Her body and mind crave the treatment because it just feels right. It feels so nice to release the restrictions that develop over the period of a day.

Educate the patient about the amount of stress and strain caused in the body every day just by doing normal activities such as sitting, driving, using the computer, and lifting. Treating every day helps to deter minor aches and pains from developing into major ones. Daily selftreatment also gives the patient time to process whatever mental stress may have occurred during the day. It becomes a time to just "chill out" and do something good for herself.

So, do they need to do this forever? Only if they want to be able to function at their optimal level and pain free for the rest of their life.

22
What about diet and supplements and JFBMFR?

The following questions come up frequently. What diet will help the JFBMFR process? Would a vegetarian diet be beneficial? Should I avoid carbohydrates? What supplements should I take?

When these questions are asked in seminars, John makes this point: it is more important to establish a system that can actually absorb nutrients than it is to put nutrients into a system that is full of restrictions. Spending money on the best supplements—or following the most recent trendy anti-aging/cleansing diet—will not do any good if the system is too restricted to process the nutrients.

Fascia goes all the way down to the cellular level; it is what gives the cell its shape. Actually, the restrictions can be preventing the nutrients from getting into the cells. The nutrients are already in the body, but the cells are clamped down and unable to process them.

Another thing to discuss is the terms "organic," "natural," and "homeopathic." Sometimes people feel using "natural" supplements means there can be no harmful side effects. Or, they believe anything "organic," "natural," or "homeopathic" is intrinsically good for them. Anything used to mask symptoms, instead of helping the body correct itself, is simply something used to treat the symptoms; it doesn't matter if it's natural or synthetic. The purity of a supplement is irrelevant when the body is unable to process the supplement due to restrictions.

If a patient is considering taking a supplement or medicine, encourage him to do his research first. Natural and organic products have just as much potential to cause side effects as do synthetic and conventional products. It's best to know about those things *before* starting to use a product. Also, suggest to the patient that he consider the training, education, experience, and expertise of the person advising him to use a product. Help the patient understand it is okay to ask questions and to think for himself.

The biggest factor in establishing and maintaining health is opening up the system. When the body is free of restrictions, it can heal itself. Until then, no matter what your patient puts in his body, it's like pouring water on a rock; nothing will be absorbed into the system.

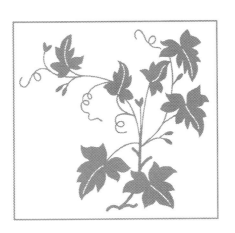

23
What about exercising?

During the treatment process, questions frequently come up about when to start exercising and what exercises to do. Of course, your answers to such questions will be based on your knowledge of exercise programs. Therapists have a variety of educational background and varying ideas of the importance of exercise. What I'm going to provide here are the basic guidelines that will coincide with your patients' progression during JFBMFR treatments.

I tell my patients to hold off on any strengthening or stabilization exercises during the beginning phases of JFBMFR. Why? Because the strengthening or stabilization exercises a patient does before her body is balanced will only further her problem. In other words, these exercises cause the patient to strengthen in a position of dysfunction.

It is very important to hold off on any trunk stabilization exercises until the pelvis is balanced and stays that way. This includes all Pilates, crunches, sit ups, etc. Many people who are really into fitness have a hard time with this idea at first. However, once a patient has felt an intense psoas release, she may be more willing to stick by this guideline!

As the patient becomes more aware of the restricted places in her body, she can start exercising *with awareness*. Suggest to the patient that when she is exercising a significantly restricted area, she should try to notice if she is strengthening or straining that area. If she is straining the area, she should either stop doing that particular exercise or perform selftreatment to that area once she is done with the exercise. This will help prevent the area from becoming more restricted.

Awareness is the key. It's all about developing communication between the mind and the body. Many people have learned to tune out or push through pain or discomfort; now, we are asking them to stop and listen. Doing this can be a very difficult at first and your patients will need your help with this concept (See chapter 9, *How do I help patients " feel under the pain"?*).

Another aspect to consider with a patient's exercise program is the reason behind the patient's need to exercise. Many people use exercise as a way to "burn off the stress." Many people have flat out said that they couldn't stop running, biking, etc. or they would "go crazy." They admit exercise is their way to deal with the stress in their lives. If they stopped exercising, then they would have to feel. Guess what, that is exactly what we want—we want them to feel! Encourage them to feel whatever it is they are trying to avoid. Then, suggest they deal with the feelings instead of stuffing them down or burning them off with exercise.

There is a difference between exercising to feel better and exercising to control feelings and emotions. Having people change or limit their exercise routine can really throw them into chaos. Talk to your patient about the need to feel and express emotions. (See chapters 16 and 17, *Why does the patient need to feel the emotions that come up?* and *What if the patient doesn't want to feel or remember that again?*)

Make sure you let your patient know she will be able to return to her exercise program. Remind her that this break is necessary to give her body time to open up and balance out. Let your patient know the goal is for her to return to the same or an even higher level of activity with less discomfort and with more ease.

Give your patients self-treatment exercises that will help release those specific tight areas which either prevent exercise or cause further tightening. This way your patients will take an active role in their recovery process and in returning to exercise. The more proactive your patients are in their healing, the more quickly they will progress.

24

Can JFBMFR help prevent surgery?

Some people arrive at our treatment center having been told surgery is the only way to improve their condition. Many of these same people have already had multiple, unsuccessful surgeries and want to avoid repeating that experience. People also call to ask if JFBMFR can prevent the need for surgery. The answer is the same to everyone: If the situation is an emergency, get the surgery! If it's not an emergency, try JFBMFR first. What have you got to lose?

No one can know before treatment whether JFBMFR will prevent the need for nonemergency surgery. However, during or after treatment, it is not unusual to find the pain, restricted motion, or other symptoms have subsided or disappeared completely and such surgery is no longer needed. This scenario is most frequent with conditions in which doctors are unable to determine the source of the pain or other symptoms, but they "think surgery should help."

Having JFBMFR treatment before nonemergency surgery can help in a couple of ways. First, treatment may help decrease the pain. Pain often occurs because the body is being compressed. Remember, a fascial restriction can have the tensile strength of up to 2000 pounds of per square inch. A force of this strength can literally crush structures in the body, producing almost every symptom in the body, including nerve and joint pain.

Second, having treatment will help open up the body, and the more open the body is before surgery, the faster the recovery. Most people have tightness and restrictions *prior* to surgery. With the effects of new scar tissue formed *after* surgery, the body becomes even tighter, and this can make recovery from surgery even more painful and difficult. Eliminating tightness and restrictions before surgery can help tissue heal much more quickly.

Joint replacement is a prime example of the kind of nonemergency surgery I've just described. Think of this situation in terms of your car needing a frontend alignment. If your car's tires are wearing unevenly, you know the alignment is off. If you just replace the tires without fixing the alignment, the new tires will just wear unevenly again. So, it makes sense to bring the car into alignment before installing new tires. Actually, having JFBMFR prior to a joint replacement may eliminate the need for the joint replacement. After treatment, if the patient still needs the replacement, his body will be in alignment. This will help the new joint last longer and help him heal with fewer problems. (As an example of how much force restrictions can cause, imagine the pressure—and the misalignment it causes—that wears out the metal components comprised by an artificial joint!)

Why not try JFBMFR first? It can't hurt and your patient has only some restrictions to lose!

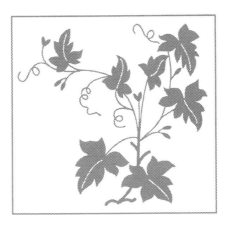

25
Should I allow family members or friends in the treatment room?

To enable a patient to benefit fully from the treatment process, we generally discourage having the patient's family members or friends in the treatment room during treatments. It can be very hard to let go completely when a family member or friend is in the room. Belief systems might be limiting the patient's healing and sometimes such belief systems were created by family dynamics. Under some circumstances, it may be appropriate to allow a family member to observe treatment to see what is involved in the process. This is generally only when a minor is being treated. In such cases, you should work to establish treatment as soon as possible without the family member present.

Each patient needs to have her treatment held as sacred space, without any fear of judgment. Some aspects of a patient's signs and symptoms may be tied into something involving her family or friends, or into an area of her life which she does not feel comfortable sharing with her family members or friends. In such cases, the patient may feel very uneasy letting go while a family member or friend is in the room. The patient might not even be aware she is holding back until she has the chance to be alone.

Make sure you are very thorough in explaining the JFBMFR process to a patient's family members or friends. Be sure to explain the benefits of the patient having the treatment session alone. To help family members and friends better understand JFBMFR, try suggesting they watch John's video *The Fireside Chat* or read his book-*Healing Ancient Wounds: The Renegade's Wisdom.*

Creating a healing environment for the patient is the first and foremost essential of providing treatment. This is a healing process and the treatment room needs to be a place considered safe. Some people may be able to look back into their adolescence and say they would have been comfortable releasing emotions or unwinding with their parents in the treatment room. However, many people do not feel this way; instead, they feel they would have been guarded and unable to release fully.

If you are a male treating a female and there is a legality issue, protect yourself by having a female staff member assist with the treatment. Do whatever you can to make sure the patient can have an open environment for healing.

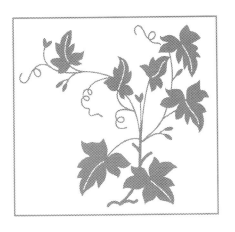

26

Why does John say, "Don't have a treatment plan."?

The medical profession as a whole has been taught to compartmentalize the body. Compartmentalization not only separates the body into parts (and associated conditions like low back strain, neck pain, shoulder tendonitis), but also separates mind and body completely. This approach tries to make "healing" a logical and linear (i.e., left brain) process: Symptom A + Symptom B = Diagnosis C.

But, as we've all found out, the body isn't linear and it can't be compartmentalized. What diagnoses does the medical profession give to those who don't fit into the box? Some examples are: fibromyalgia, chronic fatigue syndrome, and myofascial pain syndrome. Medical professionals sometimes tell a patient that part of the problem is in the patient's head. Instead of getting help with resolving the cause of their problems, patients are given pills that help decrease their symptoms but also cause them to live in a medicineinduced fog.

For example, in physical therapy school (as in most medical schools) we are taught protocols and treatment plans for each diagnosis. We are taught that if we follow these plans, we will be able to fix the problem. This keeps us in the mindset of "fixing" others, keeps us in the left brain. The truth is we need to forget about the formulas and treat each person as a unique individual. We need to enter each session like we are looking at that person for the first time. People are fluid and constantly changing. At the time of evaluation, a patient may have been rotated to the right in the pelvis. At the time of treatment, that patient might present with a rotation to the left. If you go into a treatment operating on how a patient presented at some time in the past, you won't be treating the patient's current needs.

If you go into the treatment room with a plan, you are treating with a formula or treating statistics. What you ought to do is look at the person, note what presents itself, and trust your intuitive side (i.e., the right brain). Think back to the standing evaluations you did in MFR I. Soften your focus and see where the person is being pulled. That's searching for the cause instead of treating the symptoms. Take your ego out of the treatment. We don't "fix" anyone; we are facilitators. Our job is to assist the body in doing what it already knows it needs to do.

If you go into the treatment room with a plan, then you don't know what you are doing. If you want to give the patient the treatment they need, then don't have any expectations beforehand. Let yourself go in the room with the intent to do whatever that particular person needs on that day. It might be something you've done before, or you might be drawn to an area you would not have "thought" of treating. This is one of the greatest gifts of being a JFBMFR therapist: you just let yourself be guided. Anything you need to know will be revealed during the treatment. You just need to be open to receive the messages.

So, take the pressure off. Let go of the need to figure it out. Figuring it out is not important and actually will limit your treatment. It's much more important that you be grounded and present during the treatment so you can follow what the patient's body needs. If you are connected with the patient's body, it will guide you where you need to go, no matter where you start. You have all the tools you need already inside of you. You are already great. All you have to do is allow it to occur.

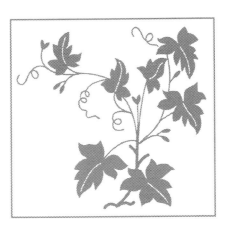

27

How do I become a better therapist?

Almost all of the therapists who come to the seminars and for the skill enhancement program have the same desire: each wants to be a "good" therapist. They often have an almost desperate look in their eyes and are full of fear that they will not be "good enough." We all want to become great overnight, and, in wanting that, put a tremendous amount of pressure on ourselves. Believe me; I know exactly what that is like!

So, here we are, trying very hard to be brilliant therapists. And of course, our traditional education taught us the results we get with our patients determine our brilliance as therapists. Based on my traditional education, I might believe that if I'm a really good therapist, I will be able to "heal" everyone! I will be like a magician, waving my wand over your body and—PRESTO—you are healed!

Then, there's John's approach. He tells us, "Take your intent out of the treatment," and "Let go of the outcome." He points out, "You can only take the patient as far as they are willing to go." And, it can be quite a surprise to hear John say, "Anyone can do what I am doing." So, you start to think, "Okay, I'm a good therapist."

But then, somewhere along the way, you find yourself in the presence of therapists who are definitely at a higher skill level. These therapists are able to help patients go into deeper places and to facilitate amazing releases. You realize that how deep a patient can go *does* have a relationship to the therapist's skill level. Having these realizations, you now know you need to take the pressure off yourself while also always striving to improve your skill level. That looks like a great example of putting one foot on the brake and one on the gas!

So, how do you become a "good" therapist?

One of main attributes of "good" therapists is they allow themselves to progress constantly along in their own healing journey. They have done the work needed to get where they are in their own healing, but they don't rest on their past experiences. They appreciate the journey they have taken thus far, and also realize there is always something more to learn, feel, or heal.

The key to becoming a "good" therapist lies in John's statement, "We can only take people as far as we've been ourselves." This *doesn't* mean we only can help people who have had traumas that are the same as our own. It *does* mean, for instance, we will not be able to provide full facilitation to a patient going through the fears and other feelings of a healing crisis if we ourselves haven't had a healing crisis and felt our own fears and other feelings. Believe me, there's a *huge* difference between talking about a healing crisis and going through one.

Does the number of JFBMFR seminars someone takes somehow equate to how "good" that person is at being a JFBMFR therapist? A person who has taken a lot of seminars has been presented with a lot of knowledge and had the opportunity for a lot of seminarbased experience. How much that person actually was able to take in—moment by moment and seminar by seminar—is an entirely different matter. A person may "get it" in the sense that they understand the benefits of JFB- MFR and can do a proper crosshand release. However, doing a technically correct crosshand release and truly connecting with a patient while performing a crosshand release are two completely different matters.

On your continued journey to become a "more skilled" therapist (you already are a good therapist!), I have the following advice:

- **Get treated often.** The more you are clear of restrictions, the more you can connect with your patients. You truly can take patients only as far as you've gone. By feeling what it's like to go through the treatment process, your advice will come from a place of knowing.

- **Understand you will always be growing.** Be gentle with yourself in your process and celebrate your successes! If you are feeling stagnant, do something about it. Get a book, go to a seminar, do something to help to put the "spirit" back into your life. In other words, become inspired (inspirited) again.

- **Pay attention to your triggers.** If you are triggered by a patient or a situation, use it as an opportunity to heal. Triggers are great guidance tools. If you wonder what you need to do to grow, just look at what triggers you!

- **Have Fun!** Most importantly, remember you are doing this to clear the junk so you can feel more love and joy! It's about living again! It's about uncovering the masterpiece inside. It's already there; all you have to do is pull off the cover!

So celebrate the therapist you have already become and keep striving to continue to learn more. Usually, when therapists first start taking the seminars and start getting treated, they do so to become better therapists. Perhaps you are, or were, one of those therapists. Eventually, you will find out you are doing it for your own benefit. Good luck and enjoy the journey!

Afterword

At his seminars, John likes to say "Life is motion" and JFB-MFR can help you regain and maintain a healthy and painfree lifestyle. I couldn't agree more, especially since it was JFB-MFR that helped give me my life back. This is why my treatment center is called Motion for Life. My hope is this book will help other people become more aware of JFB-MFR so each can get his or her life back too.

I hope this book will help you along your journey to a healthy and happy life. As more questions come up, remember you can ask them on John's chat line at: www.myofascialrelease.com. The chat line is a great resource for support and a way to connect with therapists or patients in your area.

If you have any questions, feel free to contact me through my website at www.motionforlife.net. Here's to living an active and adventurous life!